G.U. WILKINS

THE SIMPLE HEART CURE

The Ultimate Guide to Healthy Heart Remedy, Learn Everything You Need to Know About The Heart and How To Keep it Healthy and Disease-Free

Descrierea CIP a Bibliotecii Naţionale a României
G.U. WILKINS
    THE SIMPLE HEART CURE. The Ultimate Guide to
Healthy Heart Remedy, Learn Everything You Need to Know
About The Heart and How To Keep it Healthy and Disease-
Free / G.U. Wilkins. – Bucharest: Editura My Ebook, 2020
    ISBN

G.U. WILKINS

THE SIMPLE HEART CURE

The Ultimate Guide to Healthy Heart Remedy, Learn Everything You Need to Know About The Heart and How To Keep it Healthy and Disease-Free

My Ebook Publishing House
Bucharest, 2020

CONTENTS

PART TWO

HOW TO NATURALLY HAVE
A HEALTHY HEART 57

INTRODUCTION

Heart attacks are one of the leading causes of death in America. With most of us suffering from various kinds of health conditions and adding a lot of extra stress to the heart through our lack of activity and poor eating habits, it is no wonder that many of us are just ticking time bombs before we are able to experience a heart attack ourselves.

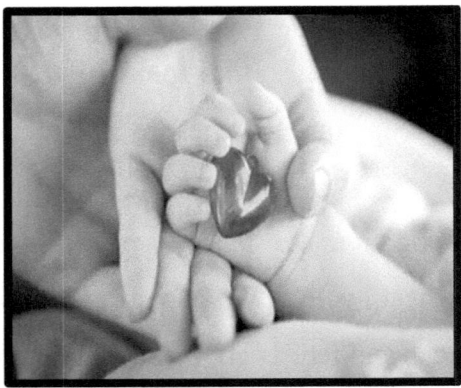

Mother Nature has taken hundreds of thousands of years of evolution to develop your heart along with the rest of your body.

Perfected by nature to become arguably the most important organ in your body. Your heart is a large muscle that pumps blood containing oxygen and other essential substances to all the organs and cells of the body. Not just that, it provides the means of removing the waste that is produced by day to day bodily functions.

This guidebook is going to spend some time looking at the various aspects of heart disease and heart attacks. You'll learn everything you need to know about heart attacks, some of the complications that arise from these, and even the risk factors that will make it more likely that you will suffer from a heart attack at some point. But the good news is there are plenty that you can do to help reduce the likelihood of the heart attack, and you just need to get started as soon as possible. In this guidebook, we are going to explore some of the things that you can do in order to keep your heart healthy and to feel good in no time.

Everyone wants to make sure that they have a strong heart and live a long, healthy life. When you are ready to prevent against heart attacks and feel as good as possible, make sure that you check out this guidebook and learn the steps that you should take to finally see results and keep your heart strong.

PART ONE

ALL ABOUT HEART ATTACKS

CHAPTER 1

WHAT IS A HEART ATTACK
OR MYOCARDIAL INFARCTION?

Heart attack occurs when there's death or necrosis of a segment of heart muscle due to the loss of blood supply. The blood supply is usually lost due to blocked coronary artery, one that provides blood to the heart muscle by blood clots. This condition is also known as coronary thrombosis.

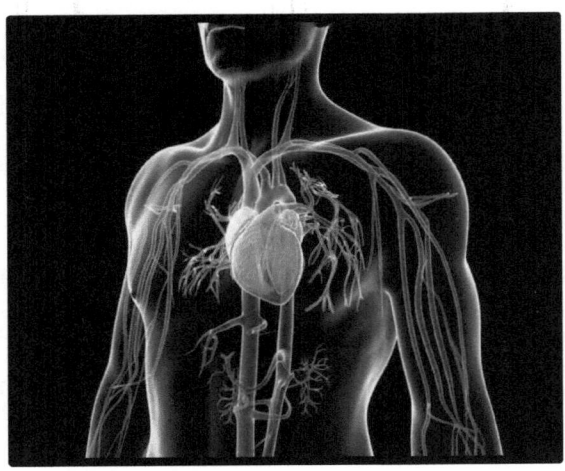

When it happens, one will experience distressing symptoms such as chest pain and electrical instability of the myocardial tissues.

Heart disease is a very general term used to describe all the different disorders and diseases that can affect your heart and its operation. One of the most common causes is oxygen starvation; this is usually the result of a blockage in the arteries that carry the flow of oxygen- rich blood from the lungs to the heart. This condition can lead to heart damage and if left untreated, the damaged heart will undergo necrosis. In other words, the heart cells will start to die. Often times, this condition is caused by a buildup of a waxy substance known as plaque.

As plaque builds up inside your arteries, it can result in the coronary (or heart) arteries being partially or totally blocked. This condition is known as atherosclerosis. This will restrict blood flow to your organs and tissues. If this condition is not treated quickly, the areas of the heart that rely on this artery will die. The once healthy heart tissues will also undergo fibrosis, forming scars that impede the usual functions of the heart. Sometimes, such condition will go off radar and difficult to be discovered. So if you leave it as it is for a long time, many heart health problems will arise in the long-term.

Symptoms of a Heart Attack or MI

With so many people suffering from heart attacks, many people are looking for ways in order to prevent these heart attacks. But before that, we should learn the early warning signs and symptoms of a heart attack or MI.

The symptoms of a heart attack can vary widely. For instance, you may have only minor chest pain while some else has excruciating pain.

Some typical heart attack symptoms for men and women are:

- Feeling of heaviness, pain, pressure, and even discomfort inside of the chest, below the breastbone, or in the arm.
- Discomfort that radiates to the back, arm, throat, or jaw.
- Feeling indigestion, fullness, and even a choking feeling. It may feel like heartburn sometimes.
- Dizziness, vomiting, nausea, and sweating.
- Extreme shortness of breath, anxiety, or weakness.
- Collapse or lose consciousness.

How to Diagnose a Heart Attack or MI?

There are thousands of people every year who fall prey to heart attacks without even realizing that they have it in the first place. They act as if nothing has happened because most who had early stages of heart attacks are asymptomatic until the crisis happens.

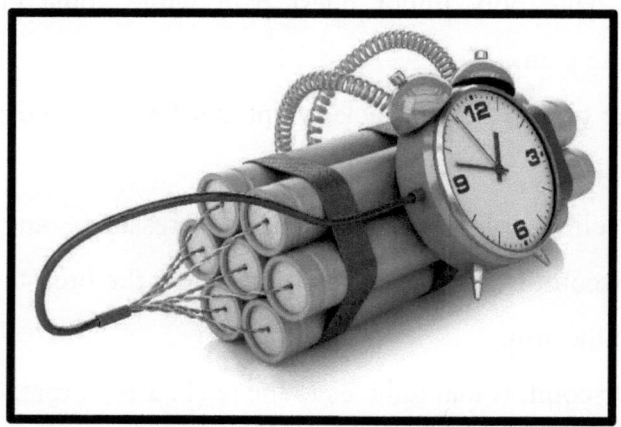

Think of it as a walking time bomb. To identify any diseases, we look at the symptoms a person is suffering from. Such symptoms for heart attack differs from one person to another. They can be mild or grave. Also, the severity and susceptibility of contracting the disease depend on the age, sex, presence of risk factors or underlying diseases. For instance, those who have diabetes usually demonstrate subtle or unusual symptoms.

In any case, if you find yourself suffering from any heart attack symptoms, you must get emergency treatment immediately. The speed of treatment is of utmost importance when dealing with episodes of heart attacks. In fact, the faster the emergency treatment, the higher the chance of survival.

When you're having an attack, bear in mind to seek help from others. Do not attempt to drive or walk yourself to the hospital when you're in excruciating pain as you'll only exacerbate the symptoms and inviting further complications. Get someone to call for an ambulance and seek prompt medical attention. Every second counts and by seeking early medical care, you can prevent further injuries to your heart tissues and even stay alive!

Chest Pain – Cardiogenic VS Non-Cardiogenic

Most people experience chest pain to some degree, at one time or another over the course of their lives. This is often caused by anxiety because chest pain is so often associated with heart disease. Fortunately, almost all chest pain has little to do with the heart, but it is not something you should ignore.

Understanding the difference between the different types of chest pain helps in diagnosing heart diseases. Pain in the left part of the chest is one of the earliest signs a person can have to pinpoint the disease. The next step is to determine whether the pain originates from the heart or other factors.

The chest and lung areas are made up of many different structures all of which can produce pain. The most common type of pain or tenderness is in the muscles and bone joints around the chest. The lining or pleura around the lungs can be associated with pain if it becomes inflamed or irritated, but the lungs do not contain any of the nerve connections that will induce the feelings of pain.

The esophagus or the tube from your mouth to your stomach is another area in your chest that can give you pain. Heartburn, as it is often referred to or refluxing has nothing to do with your heart, but can often give a pain that feels like a heart disorder. The esophagus can also have or give spasms, which is also non- cardiogenic.

Cardiac or heart-related chest pain is more often experienced in the morning. Symptoms include a dull, constricted pressure with burning or squeezing sensation. Instead of

18

superficial pain, people usually find that the pain comes from the deeper areas of their chest. However, it can be difficult when it comes to describing the location of the pain.

It may feel like the pain originates from all areas such as back, neck, head, and throat or even from the arms (often the left upper arm). Not knowing where the pain comes from, people commonly described that "the pain came out of nowhere." Chest pain is often brought on by some form of exertion like carrying a heavy bag, sweeping or digging.

Extreme temperature while exercising or working can also cause a heart attack. It can also follow after eating a heavy meal, then doing physical work. These types of pain usually last as long as the physical activity you are doing continues, but in most cases reduces quite quickly once the activity that brought it on is stopped.

Some forms of heart-related pain, such as angina, can be aggravated by lying down, but standing or sitting and even leaning into the discomfort area can help to relieve it.

If you feel these types of discomfort or pain, then it is very important to seek medical help immediately. Other types of chest pain that are not related to the heart most often manifest in or towards the end of the day. The pain often feels much sharper and is usually in one area that can be identified easily. This type of pain normally occurs without any real warning or specific reason apart from doing an unusual activity.

Heartburn may develop after eating oily or high carbohydrate foods. Often these types of pain come and go quickly, sometimes lasting only a few seconds or minutes, at other times they may remain for several hours. Simple exercises, especially breathing exercises will often help relieve or stop this type of pain. It will usually respond well to analgesics such as aspirin and heat packs.

What your Medical Professional Will Do

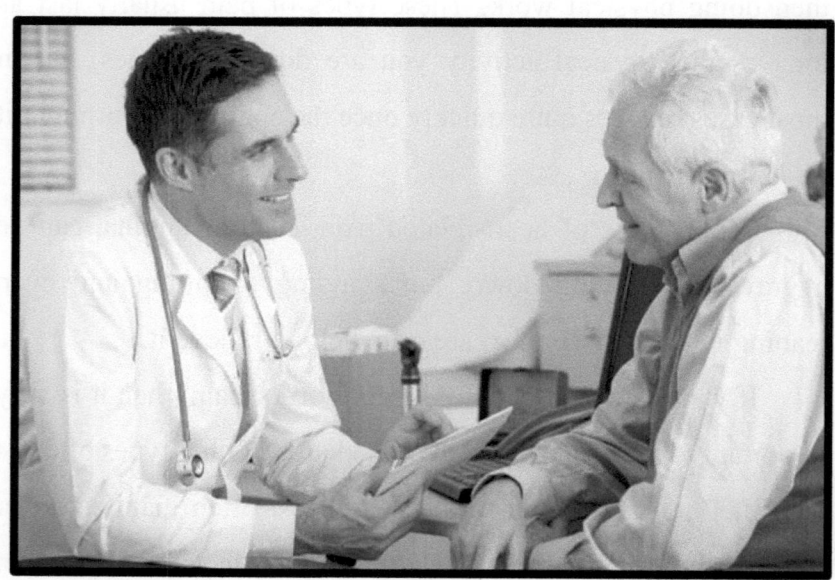

Your health professional will usually ask you a series of questions such as your age and sex; your eating habits and your physical history. They will take your vital signs such as weight, blood pressure, temperature and may do a test to determine your body fat ratio.

If you are a 25 year old gymnast or martial arts student who has just started lifting weights and doing a body building course, then it is safe to assume that your pain is muscular in origin.

If you happen to be a 56 year old male who is a heavy smoker and drinker as well as someone who does little physical work, a high- stress job and also has high blood pressure, eats mainly processed foods as well as having a family history of heart disease; then it is safe to assume that your health professional is going to be looking for a heart-related reason for your pain. This is because all these factors contribute to an increased risk of heart attack.

You will probably be asked to undergo a variety of tests and possible chest X-ray to find out what your problem is and find out what's best for you.

In case you've determined that the chest pain is due to the diseased heart, seek emergency aid as quickly as possible. Early detection of the root of the problem can help you prevent further attacks and even put an end to heart attacks. By providing early treatment, you'll have the best chance for a full or satisfactory recovery over the shortest timeframe possible.

CHAPTER 2

COMPLICATIONS OF A HEART ATTACK

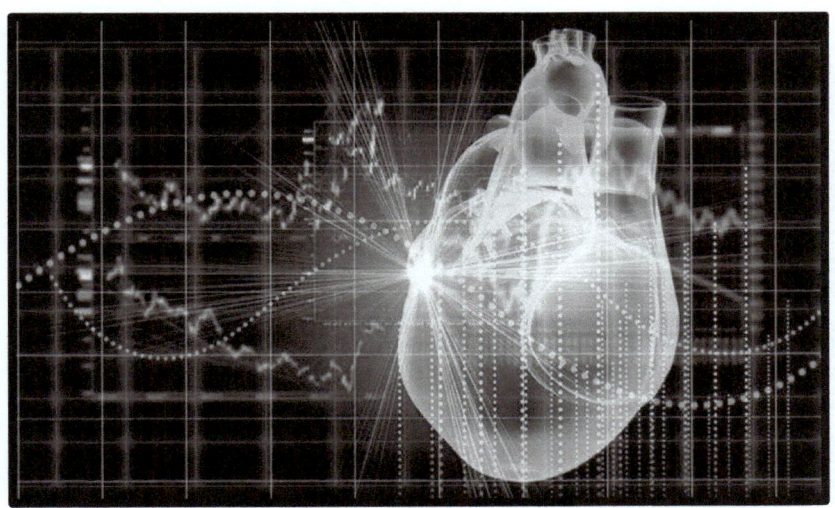

Heart Failure

Heart failure occurs when your heart is unable to pump enough blood around your body to meet all your bodily needs. Heart failure can cause many complications to all the body organs and parts. Areas such as the brain, lungs, kidneys, skin and nervous system can be affected. The veins in the arms and hands, legs and feet, abdomen and neck can also be affected, often becomes swollen. Heart failure can also cause shortness of breath, especially when you're doing physical work.

Valvular Heart Disease

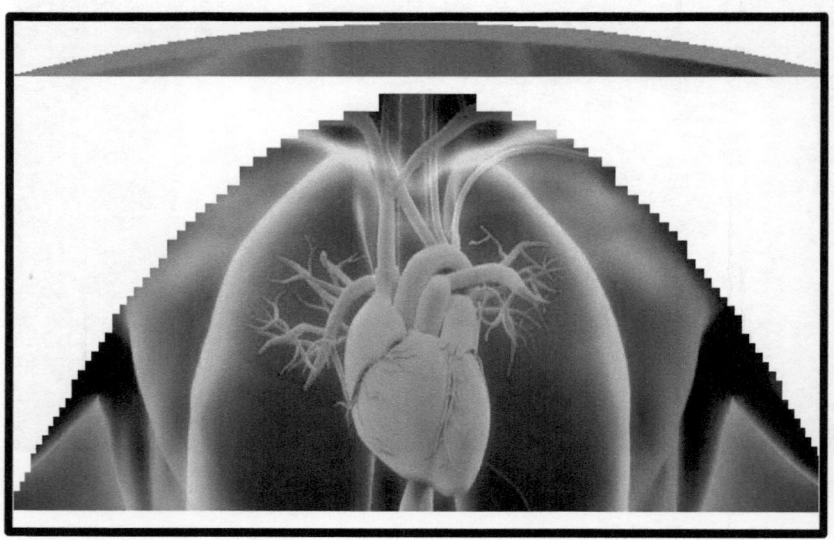

This condition is where the valves in your heart that control the free flow of blood are not working properly. The valves of the heart ensure that your blood freely flows in a forward direction and cannot leak backward. The way in which a healthy heart operates is the same for everyone.

The heart contains four chambers with the heart valves placed at the exit of each chamber. The blood flows through both your right and left atria into the ventricles through the mitral and tricuspid valves. When your ventricle chambers are full, the valves will shut, stopping the blood from returning to the atria when the ventricles contract. When the ventricles start to contract, the aortic and pulmonic valves are forced to open. The blood from the left ventricle goes into the aorta and then to the rest of the body after passing through the aortic valve. The blood from the right ventricle goes into the pulmonary artery through the pulmonic valve.

Once the ventricles are done contracting and begin to relax, both the valves are shut. This prevents any blood from flowing back. This process repeats itself throughout an entire lifetime. There are two main types of heart valve disease.

Valvular stenosis occurs when one or more valves are narrowed, stiffened, thickened or blocked. It can lead to the heart pump insufficiency, and there'll be a lack of blood on different body parts. All four of the heart valves can develop stenosis.

The other common type is valvular insufficiency. This happens when a heart valve does not seal or close properly, allowing some blood to be forced or leak back into the chamber. If this condition worsens, it forces the heart to work harder to supply the needed blood to the body.

Some forms of heart valve disease are congenital while some may only be detected later in infancy. Other forms can develop during a person's lifetime. However, the cause is still unknown, but it's definitely linked to inadequate diets and sedentary lifestyles. This form of the condition usually affects the pulmonic or aortic valves. Sometimes, they can have defective leaflets that are deformed, incorrect size or not attached properly.

Sometimes, people are born with bicuspid aortic valve disease; this is where there are only two leaflets instead of three. As a result, the valves are unable to open or close properly or tightly. Acquired valve disease occurs when valves that were normal at birth and in early life have changed or developed complications.

It can happen for a variety of reasons, mainly infections or diseases, including rheumatic fever (caused by an untreated bacterial infection such as strep throat). Often times, when this type of congenital disease is left untreated, it can quickly lead to inflammation of the heart valves. Another heart valve disease is known as endocarditis, this occurs when harmful bacteria enters the blood stream and then attacks the heart valves. It usually results in holes and growths developing as well as subsequent scarring. This bacterium is often able to enter the blood stream because of IV drug use, dental procedures, surgery, or severe infections.

Another common condition is called Mitral valve prolapse. This is a condition that is known to affect about 1.5% of the general population. This condition causes the leaflets of the mitral valve to move back into the left atrium when the heart contracts. As a result, the heart tissues will become stretchy, and leaking will most likely occur at the valves. Normally this condition does not become problematic and does not require treatment unless there are other complications.

Another thing that can affect the heart valves are some sexually transmitted diseases such as syphilis. Besides that, high blood pressure and many types of drugs can also cause heart valves deformities.

Cardiogenic Shock

Cardiogenic shock occurs whenever there's sudden failure of pump action of the heart in supplying enough oxygen-rich blood to the organs of your body. Statistics show that about 50%

of people who develop this condition will survive if immediate help is available.

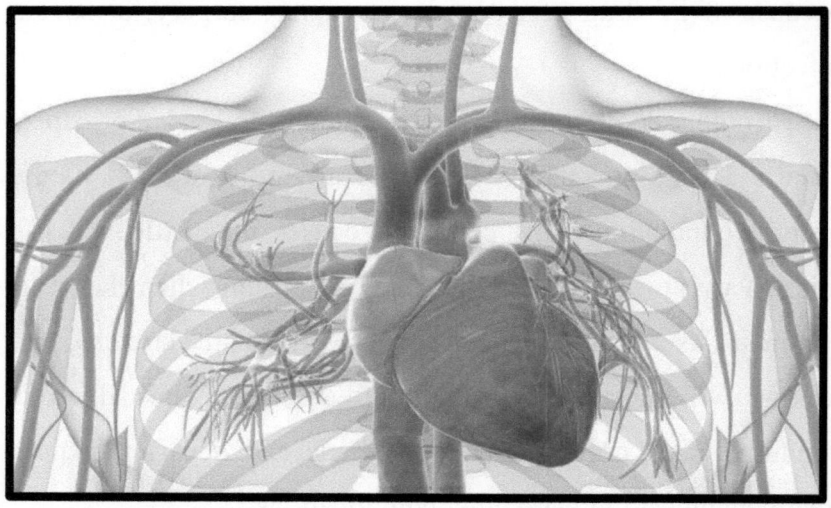

This condition is usually caused by the damage to the heart muscle. It is most common with people who are having a severe heart attack. Only about 7 to 8% of people who experience a heart attack will have a cardiogenic shock. When people die from heart attacks, it is usually due to the cardiogenic shock, not the actual heart attack.

Because of this "shock", the body has a dangerously low blood pressure. Another type of shock, hypovolemic shock is where the heart cannot pump enough blood because of blood loss usually from trauma.

Vasodilatory Shock

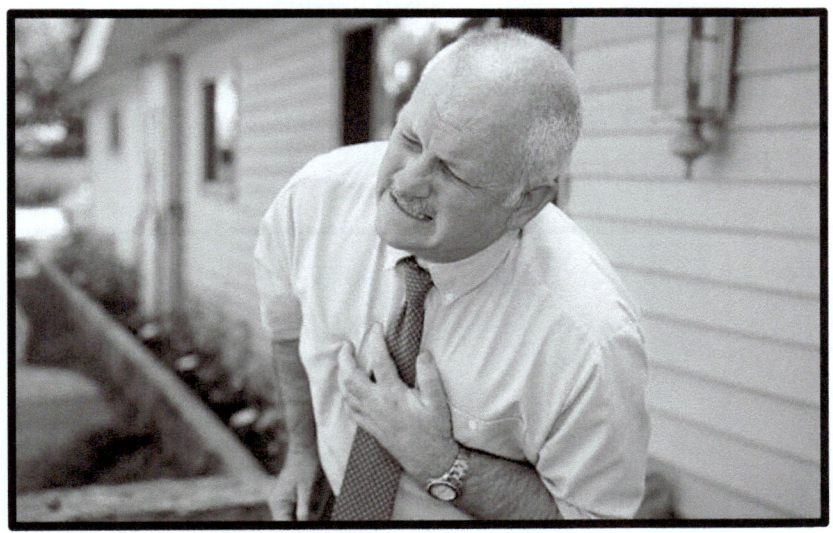

Vasodilatory shock is when the blood vessels relax abruptly, causing blood pressure to become so low that there is not enough pressure to pump the blood to areas that need it. This can be caused by a bacterial infection in the bloodstream or a severe allergic reaction to certain substances. This can also occur when the nervous system is damaged.

When someone is suffering from this type of "shock" regardless of the cause, it means not enough oxygen is reaching their vital organs. They only a few minutes before the lack of oxygen starts to do damage that is usually not repairable. If it is not treated quickly, it is likely to cause permanent organ damage or death. If you know or think that a person is in shock, call an ambulance so they can get treatment quickly.

Pulmonary Embolism

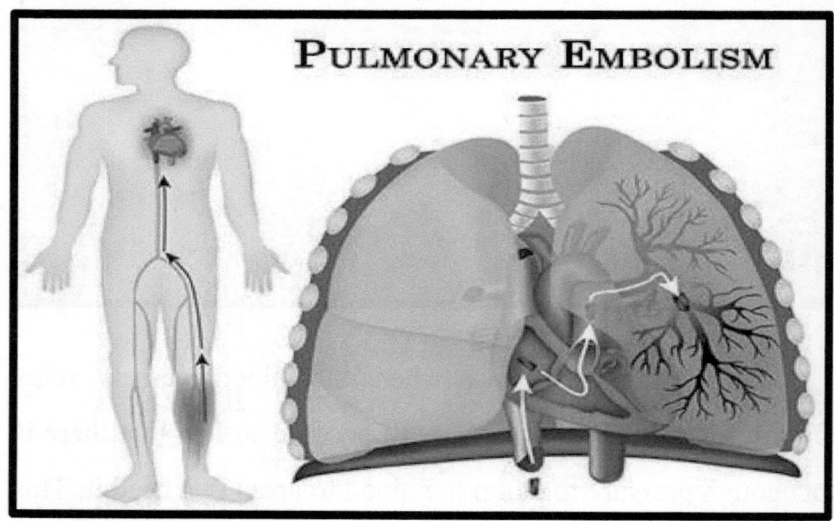

Pulmonary embolism is a blockage in the pulmonary arteries in your lungs. Usually, a pulmonary embolism is caused when blood clots from the legs and sometimes other areas of the body (deep vein thrombosis) travel to the lungs.

A pulmonary embolism can reduce or block the blood flow to the lungs, becoming a life-threatening condition. With prompt and expert treatment, the chances of this condition resulting in death are greatly reduced. One of the best ways to prevent a pulmonary embolism is to take adequate measures to prevent blood clots in your legs. If blood clots are formed, quickly eradicate them.

Arrhythmias

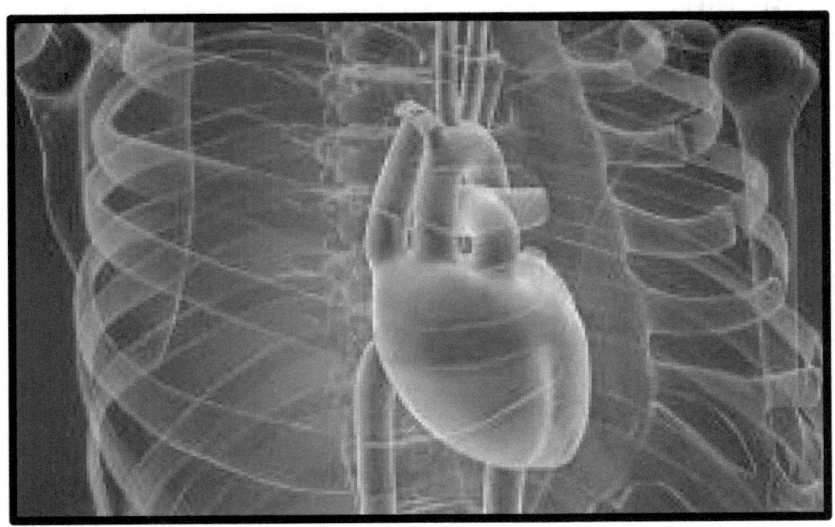

Arrhythmia is the term given to a condition where the rhythm of your heartbeat changes. This can happen when your heart rhythm is too slow, too fast or if it has an irregular rhythm. Sometimes an arrhythmia can cause your heart to just stop

31

beating, which is called "sudden cardiac arrest" or SCA. If it is not treated immediately, it can cause a loss of consciousness and death of a person.

Broken Heart Syndrome

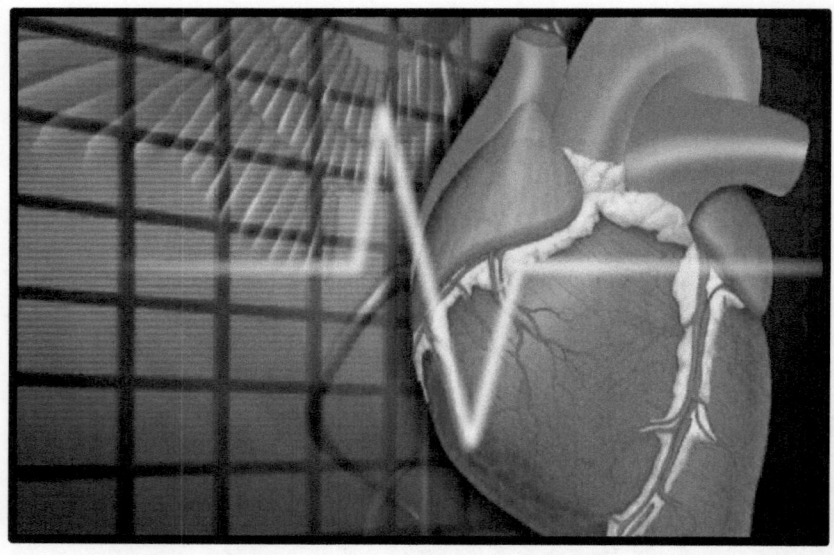

This condition is commonly triggered by emotional stress and heartaches from loss of loved ones, falling out of love, being rejected, frequent anxiety and so on. Thus, it is named as Broken heart syndrome. The most common signs of broken heart syndrome are chest pains and shortness of breath; sometimes it is accompanied by cardiogenic shock or arrhythmias.

The other symptoms of broken heart syndrome tend to differ from those of a heart attack:

- The symptoms occur abruptly after experiencing extreme physical or emotional stress
- The results of Electrocardiogram (ECG is a test to observe the heart's electrical activities) are usually different from those who have had a heart attack. For instance, those who had a heart attack in the past will show a deep Q-wave in their ECG graph
- When tested there are no signs of coronary arteries being blocked
- There is usually, unusual movement and possible ballooning of the left ventricle or lower left chamber of the heart
- The recovery time is relatively quick, often within a few days or weeks as opposed to a heart attack which usually takes a month or more

Arteries often harden as a person ages, losing their suppleness and elasticity over time. Although smoking is thought to be one of the major contributors to this condition, the actual cause remains unknown. Chemically derived drugs are believed to be another contributor along with a poor diet or a diet that contains a large amount of preservatives, artificial flavors, and colorings.

Myocardial Aneurysm

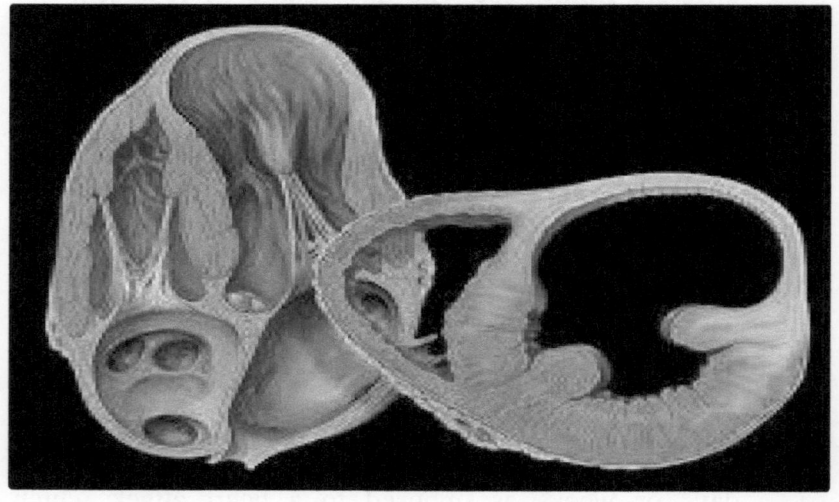

An aneurysm occurs due to weakened blood vessel, causing it to swell and fill with blood. Often these are formed after a heart attack. They often occur around the base of your septum, or in the aorta. This can cause a constriction of the blood flow to the body, resulting in heart disease. Eventually, aneurysms will be lined with scar tissue, which usually stops them from rupturing.

Aneurysms in ventricular generally grow slowly. The common symptoms are tiredness, lack of energy, and stamina. Blood clots can form inside some ventricular aneurysms, which can lead to serious complications and even death. Death is common when the blood clots break away and spread throughout the blood stream.

Some aneurysms are congenital while others are caused by a heart attack. The blood clots formed around them can block the blood vessels, resulting in restricted movement and tissue death in a limb, a stroke, ventricular aneurysm or arrhythmia.

CHAPTER 3

EMERGENCY CARE

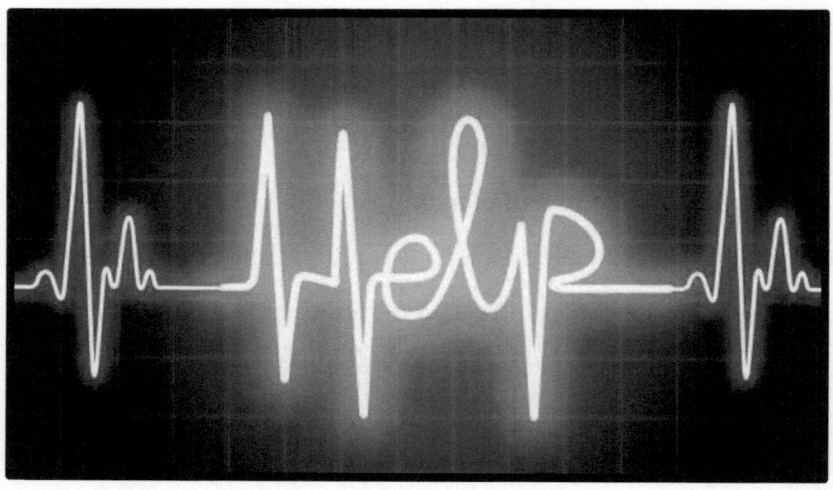

Often times, there won't be obvious signs of pre-heart attack. This disease is usually asymptomatic until the later stage. Early signs of Heart Attack include feeling pain or discomfort on his or her chest and shoulders, tiredness, lack of energy, breathing difficulty, and so on.

Complaints might differ for each person, but when heart attack actually happens, one would experience sharp pain on his or her left chest for at least 15 minutes. Men and women have different symptoms. For instance, women usually do not experience any chest pain; their common symptoms are fatigue, disturbed sleep patterns, shortness of breath, indigestion and anxiety issues.

If you think you have heart attack, call emergency services right away. Do not wait, as every minute counts. A patient's chances of full recovery can be drastically reduced by the delay of treatment. Call emergency services and talk a trained operator to assist you.

The 6 Signs of Heart Attack

So how do you determine whether a person is suffering from a heart attack? Here are the six signs of heart attack that you can take note of.

Heart Attack sign 1: Chest Pain or Discomfort

For men, chest discomfort is the most common symptom of a heart attack. Usually, they'll experience a tight, heavy, or burning sensation. It can also feel like indigestion or heartburn.

This sensation usually begins in the middle of the chest, and then it moves to other areas of the body. This discomfort usually come and go.

Some people experience no pain at all, just discomfort or a dull type of pain, which can grow to be quite intense; others will not have pain just discomfort.

Heart Attack sign 2: Discomfort or Pain in Other Parts of The Body

The symptoms of a heart attack can also manifest in different parts of the body, such as one or both arms, back, stomach, jaw or the neck. Different people, especially women, will experience pain or discomfort in the jaw or back during an attack.

Heart Attack sign 3: Shortness of breath

Feeling short of breath is a common heart attack symptom. It is normal for a person to experience shortness of breath after some physical work or exercise but if this happens when you're resting, it is often a sign of heart attack. It is caused by the leaking of fluid into the lungs. To unusually fatigued women, it can sometimesbe an accompanying symptom.

Heart Attack sign 4: Nausea, Sweating or Clamminess

Many people, especially women, when having a heart attack will feel nauseous, excessive sweating or clamminess. These symptoms can also be indications of the flu, but if these symptoms occur abruptly or you also have other indications of a heart attack, call the emergency services immediately.

Heart Attack sign 5: A general feeling of extreme fatigue or weakness

Sometimes, the first complaint you may hear from a heart attack patient is general weakness or fatigue. It might not sound like much, but this is a common indication that most potential heart attack patients experience prior to the attack. But this symptom alone is not enough to diagnose or expect a heart attack as there are too many causes of weakness and fatigue. It can be due to lack of oxygen, not having enough sleep, poor eating habits, anemia, arthritis, and others.

Heart Attack sign 6: Collapse or Falling

Often a person with heart attack will collapse or lose consciousness, unlike other chest condition where this rarely happens. Again, if you find someone collapses and lose consciousness, bring him or her to an open area and call for an ambulance right away.

Early Warning Signs of a Heart Attack

Heart attacks usually give a bit of a warning before they happen (except with Heartbreak Attack). Often this can happen days or in some cases months before an attack is imminent, and the heart muscle becomes damaged.

- High Blood Pressure is a sign of possible heart disease

- Chronic Heartburn can be an indication of heart problems

- Reduced cardiovascular fitness and shortness of breath

- High blood LDL cholesterol levels

- The feeling of being unwell or run-down, before a heart attack

- There are reports showing that a lot of people feel a sense of impending death before experiencing a heart attack. This is quite common and may have something to do with depression, which is also a strong indicator of heart problems.

❑ Abdominal pain and indigestion are common signs of heart attack, especially for people over 55.

Because of the similar symptoms in many different conditions or diseases, it can be hard to tell that you are experiencing a heart attack. So make sure to keep an eye out for other symptoms. The more symptoms you find, the easier it is to diagnose a heart attack. Routine checkups from your health provider are advisable for prevention and cure.

What To Do Before Help Arrives:

o Having a heart attack is a traumatic experience. Often, people will be very panic when they are having a heart attack. So try to remain calm.

o The best recovery position is when you are sitting in the "W" position; this is with the back supported at a 75 degree angle and the legs bent so the knees are up and feet flat on the ground, forming a W shape.

o Another recommended position is to lie flat on your back with your feet up above your heart, the Venus position. This opens your diaphragm; it makes breathing easier and increases the oxygen supply.

o Once the person is comfortable, all tight fitting clothing should be loosened to avoid any restriction.

o It is important that the person does not walk around; lying or sitting in a relaxed position without pressure on the lungs is the best.

o If someone is expecting a heart attack, they may be carrying aspirin or nitroglycerin. Usually, they will know the required dose. Help them to take a small amount.

o If a person's heart stops beating, it becomes necessary to start CPR, but it is important that a person administering CPR is trained correctly.

o If you do not know how to do CPR then doing heart compressions is the best option. When CPR is administered as soon as a person's heart stops beating, the person's chances of survival are drastically increased.

What To Do If You Are Having A Heart Attack When You're Alone

The first thing you should do is call emergency services, give your location first, then name and try and state your problem.

Only after you have summoned emergency services should you call others such as friends or family. The emergency service operator is trained to help in cases of emergency so follow their instructions until help arrives.

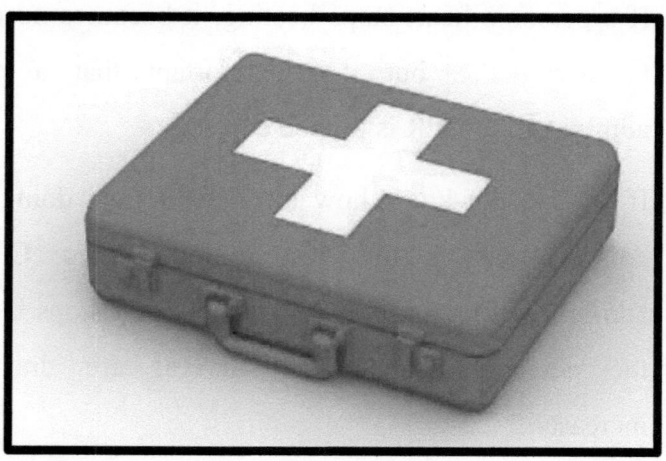

If you are completely alone and do not have a phone, there is still one thing you can do that may save your life. This self-procedure is controversial, it has been suggested that it could make matters worse if it is not done correctly. But if you are alone and there is no available help, then this is a viable option.

Take a very deep breath and then cough vigorously right from the bottom of your chest (in the same way a cat will cough to get rid of a fur ball). For this to work effectively, a person needs to take very deep breaths about every 2 seconds. Breathe in and make a deep prolonged cough. This procedure has to be maintained until your heart regains a regular rhythm and is beating normally. It is best to repeat this until help arrives.

What this procedure does is to bring large amounts of oxygen into your lungs; the coughing squeezes the heart and keeps the blood moving. This squeezing pressure on your heart, at about every 2 seconds will help your heart regain its normal rhythm. By doing so, you should be able to remain in a stable condition while waiting for help to arrive.

CHAPTER 4

RISK FACTORS FOR HEART DISEASE

One of the best ways for you to ensure that you aren't going to suffer from heart disease or heart attacks is to understand some of the risk factors for heart disease. There are many risk factors that you do not have any control over such your family history and age. But there are certain factors that you have full control of in order to prevent heart problems or a heart attack. For example, to reduce the risk of heart attack, you can change your diet, lifestyle and attitude.

- **Genetic or Family History**

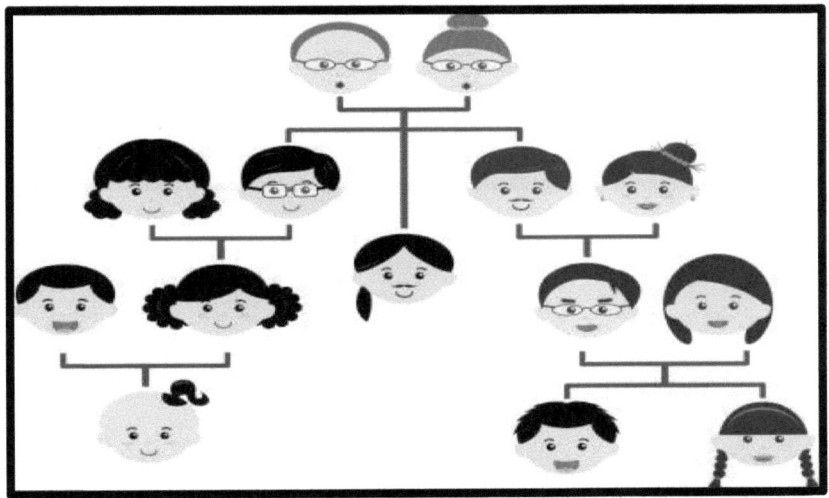

If you have a family history of people with heart disease, this can increase your chances of developing a similar type of condition. With the combination of heredity and unhealthy life choices such as eating unhealthy foods and smoking, the risk of heart disease can increase even more. If you take the necessary steps to look after your heart, you can reduce the chances of developing all forms of heart disease.

After menopause, some women are more likely to develop heart problems. It is because at this stage of their life, they are producing less estrogen. Hence, to reduce the risk of heart disease, they need to vary their diet accordingly.

- **Obesity and its Effects**

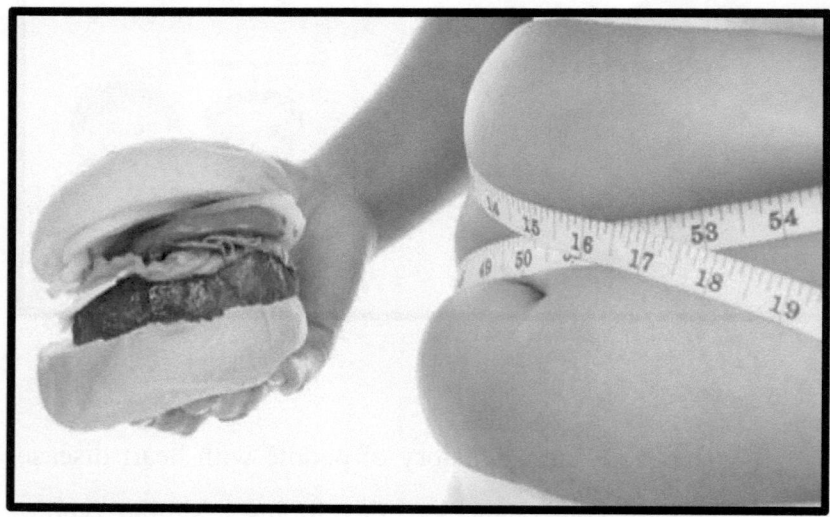

Obesity is a growing global health problem. Someone who is obese has four times the likelihood of developing heart diseases. Furthermore, those with a family history of high blood pressure or diabetes will have a greater risk for heart disease.

Obesity is now recognized as an inflammatory disease; it is often thought to be a symptom or indication of other conditions a person may have. Not as it used to be considered, just an eating disorder. Different studies have confirmed that obesity is a major contributor to causing heart disease and heart attacks.

- **Poor Diet, The wrong foods, Clogged Heart Vessels – Strokes**

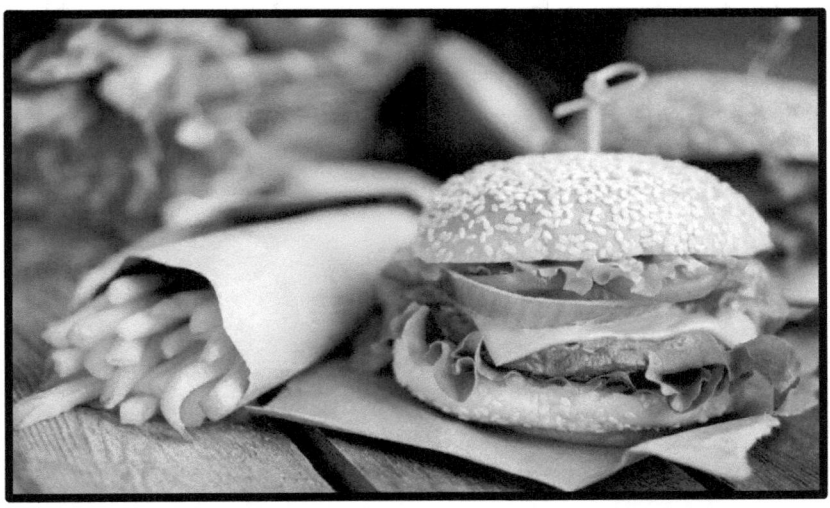

There is absolutely no doubt that having a poor diet or a diet that is deficient in many vital nutrients is a leading contributor to the extremely high incidences of heart disease that have become a reality for many people today.

Our foods have been stripped of a significant portion of their natural goodness by processing and the synthetic methods used to grow them. Processed salt, highly refined grains, high fructose corn syrup and refined vegetable oils are the four "poisons" that are found in most of our diets. The combination of these, clog up the arteries and blood vessels of the lungs and heart causing heart disease.

- **Smoking**

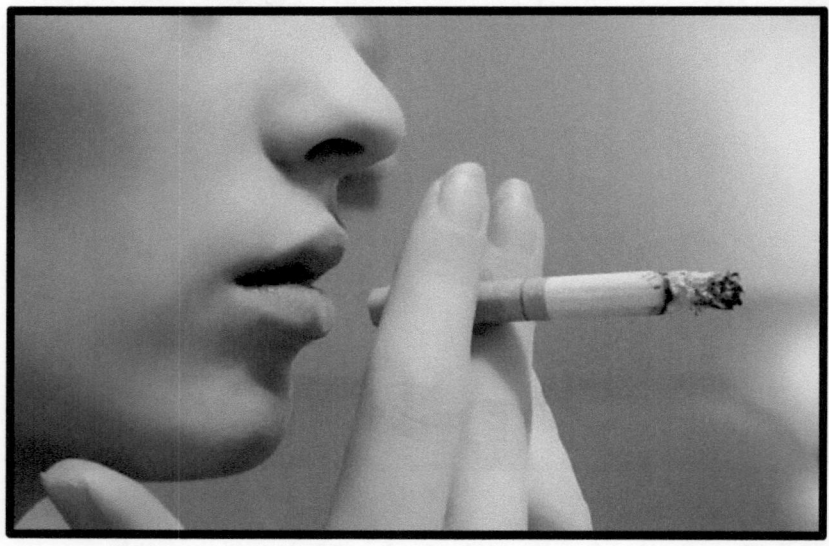

Everyone is aware that smoking is likely to damage your lungs, but many do not seem to realize that it is also a major risk factor for heart disease. In fact about one in every five people who die from a heart attack because of smoking. If you smoke, you are at least four times more likely to get heart disease than non- smokers. And the risks are even higher for women who take birth control pills.

Secondhand smoke exposure is also a risk factor for having a heart attack. The nicotine in cigarette smoke reduces the oxygenation of your blood. As a result, the amount of oxygen your lungs can send to your heart will be significantly reduced. It also leads to high blood pressure and increased heart rate due to the compensation mechanism that your body triggered when it's deprived of oxygen. Nicotine is also known to harm the inner walls of blood vessels and arteries, and also forms unwanted blood clots.

- **Drinking**

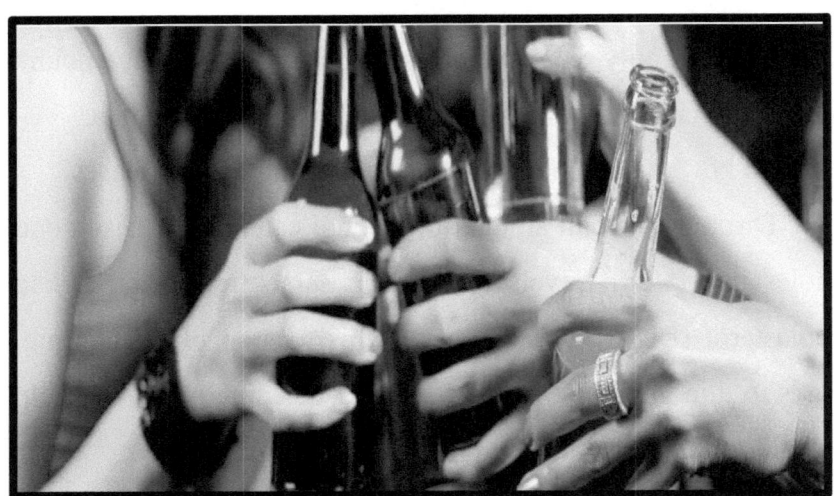

Consuming a small amount of alcohol can benefit our health. Examples of health benefits are:

- Preventing heart diseases
- Lowers the risk of developing ischemic stroke (Which occurs when your coronary arteries are blocked or narrowed, resulting in decreased blood supply)
- Possibly reduce your risk of diabetes

However, doctors will never advise heart patients to drink alcohol in any case. It's because 90% of the patients who're allowed to drink alcohol won't be able to control themselves! Instead of drinking a little, they end up chugging down the whole bottle, especially chronic alcoholics.

You can only reap the benefits by drinking a small amount, any more than that the recommended volume is detrimental.

So how does alcohol helps in preventing heart diseases?

Drinking a small amount of alcohol can help to raise good cholesterol (HDL) levels and at the same time reduces bad cholesterol (LDL) levels. It also helps to stop blood clotting, tends to thin the blood, allow for easier bleeding and could help to hold off a heart attack, but only if used in moderation.

- **High Cholesterol**

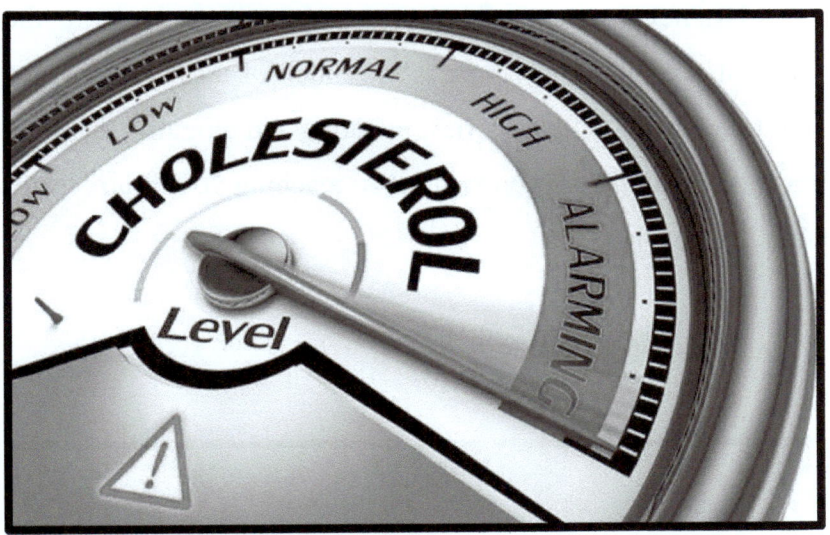

Cholesterol has been blamed for heart disease for many years, but it is now known that cholesterol is in fact healthy. In fact, it's one of the most important substances the body produces. After all, the body needs cholesterol to carry out its functions. For instance, our brain and liver are made of good cholesterol.

Our body can produce cholesterol on its own. However, the problem arises when we consume too much 'bad' cholesterol, also known as LDL or low-density lipoproteins. Eating processed sugars, hydrogenated vegetable oils and too much omega-6 fatty acids causes an oversupply of LDL.

LDL helps to carry cholesterol around our body to the areas that need it. When there is too much of it, the excess can cling to the walls of the arteries, irritating and clogging them up, preventing enough oxygen-rich blood reaching your brain, heart, and other organs.

- **Diabetes**

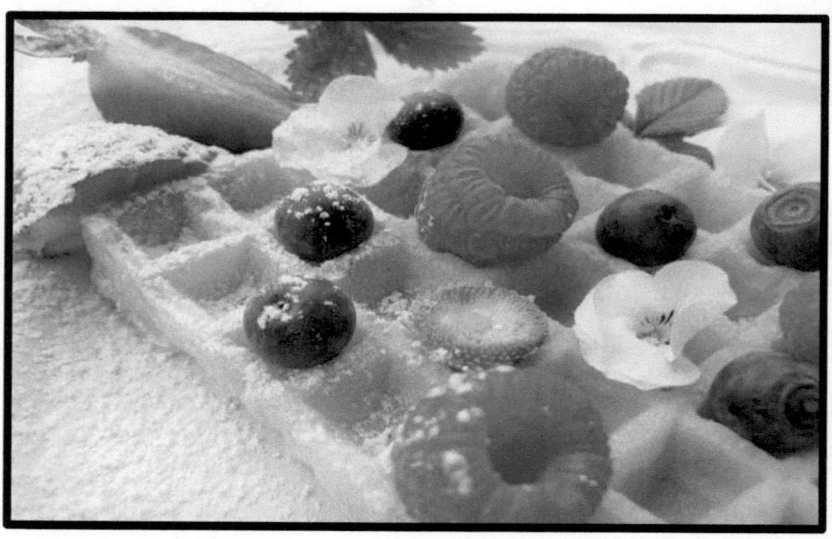

People with diabetes tend to have a high blood glucose level, which can damage your blood vessels and the nerves that control the blood vessels in your heart in the long-term.
54

Many people with diabetes can develop heart disease at a young age, and those with diabetes are almost twice as likely to have heart failure as non-diabetics.

As with all heart conditions, if you take the proper steps to manage your diabetes, your risk factors will be substantially reduced.

- **Physical Activity**

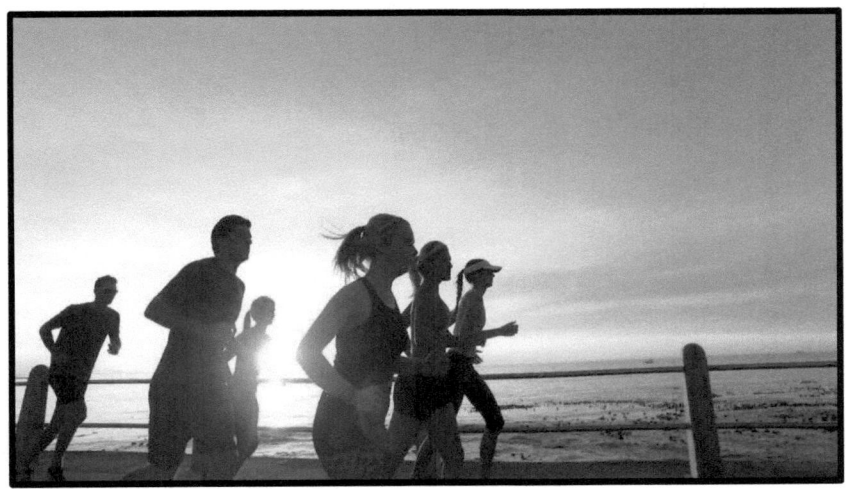

Doing very little or no physical activity is a major cause of heart disease and heart attacks. This is because they cannot burn up the excess calories, which results in fat tissues formation.

The body is designed to perform a certain amount of activity daily to keep it supple, healthy and function properly.

When the body takes in more food or energy than it needs over an extended period, this will lead to obesity, which can result in many diseases. The body needs exercise to stay in peak condition, which is a good way to train a heart health.

PART TWO

HOW TO NATURALLY HAVE A
HEALTHY HEART

Taking proper care of your heart is like finding a fountain of youth. It's a no-brainer that if you look after your heart, you will live a long and healthy life. Most people require 7 to 8 hours of quality sleep a night to maintain a healthy heart, as this is the time for self-repair as well as to maintain healthy heart arteries.

If your blood pressure is too high, it can cause damage to artery walls, resulting in scar tissues formation and loss of flexibility. This situation can make it harder for oxygen-rich blood to get to your heart and other organs. The harder the heart has to work continually, the quicker it can wear out. Therefore, it is important to maintain a healthy blood pressure.

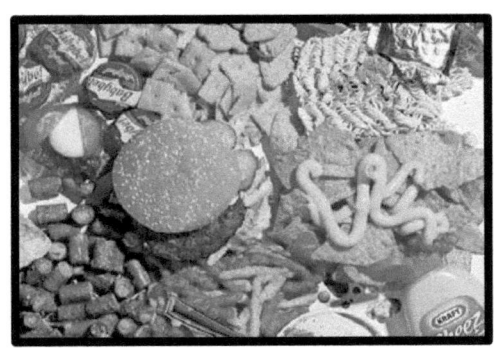

Pay attention to your diet and avoid as many processed foods as possible. At the same time, remember to perform as much physical exercise as possible.

The human heart works best if you provide good quality clean fuel, in other words, fresh, wholesome organic food and minimal processed foods.

Also, choose healthier drinks such as fruit juices or plain water instead of soft drinks to improve your overall health. Try to balance your work and home life. Spend more time with your family, friends and loved ones. This practice is good for both your mental and physical health. Check your vital signs with regular check-ups to maintain a healthy heart.

CHAPTER 5

LIFESTYLE CHOICES FOR A STRONG, HEALTHY HEART

There comes a time in everyone's lives when we have to decide and commit to making healthy lifestyle changes. Often times, it's when they realize that their body is starting to break down, in the terminal stage of a disease, or experience the pain of losing a loved one from ill health. These situations are often the turning point in their lives where they finally decide on the best course for them and their family.

It's always better to live a healthy life, full of vitality, youth, and vibrancy than to live a sick life that constantly relies on health support. Our environment plays a significant role in our heart health. So if your living condition is not conducive to your health, such as living in a heavily polluted area with poor hygiene and health facilities, the best option is to relocate to somewhere else.

Diet: The Importance of a Healthy Diet

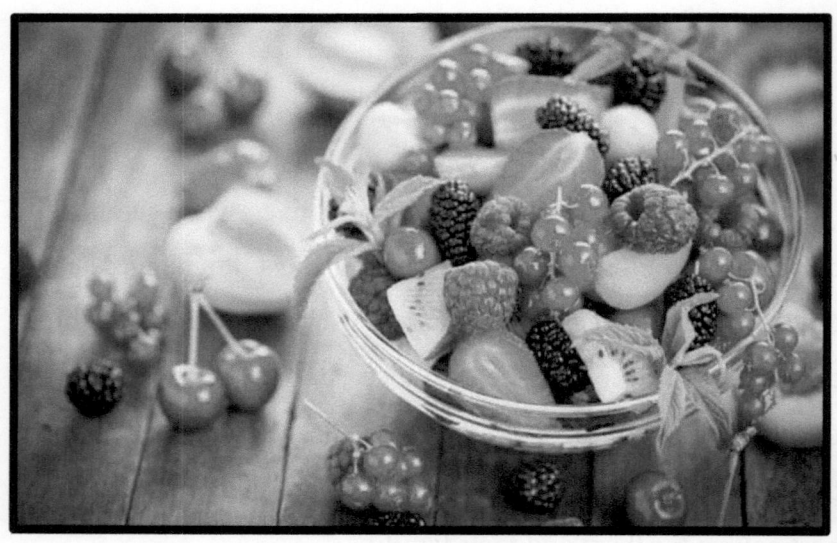

Our bodies and hearts form an extremely complex organic living machine, but far more advanced than anything a man can create. But like all machines, it needs the right fuel and lubrication to maintain it. Have you heard of the saying that "Your body is your vehicle for this life's journey"? Thus, you should honor your body more than anything else. Think about it, would you put cheap vegetable oil in your new car or try and fill the tank with cheap, dirty old fuel.

Then why would you do that to your body, you can always buy a new car, but you cannot get a new body (well, maybe a new heart, but what a hassle and expense). Surely it is sensible to only use the very best fuels for your body! Of course, what I meant by fuel is your diet intake. Only choose the food that'll benefit your health, not destroy your body.

Exercise - The best Heart Exercises

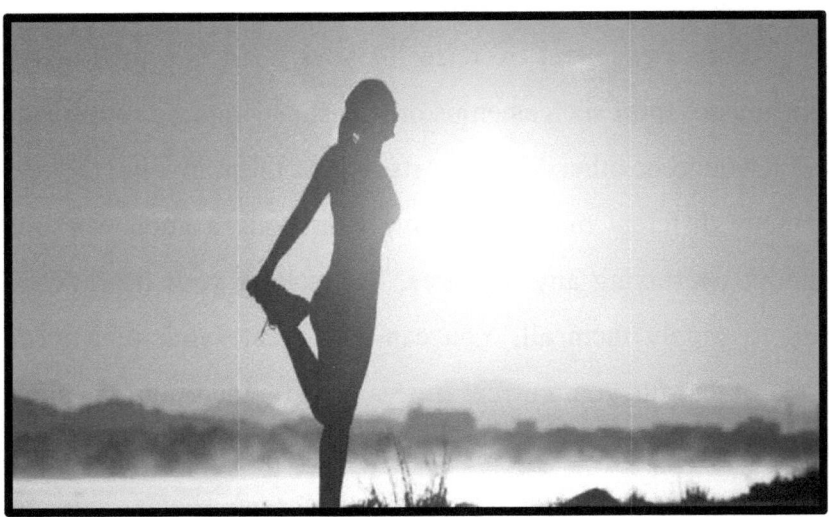

So what is the best and most effective exercise for preventing heart diseases? Studies show that high-intensity exercise coupled with slightly longer periods of active recovery is not only beneficial to your heart's health, but also aids in weight loss, diabetes, and improving your overall fitness level.

It can be done by walking for 3 minutes at your normal speed and then walking 1 minute at a brisk pace. By raising and lowering your heart rate continuously through simple high-intensity workouts, you can have a better vascular function, burn more calories, and also enhance the body's detoxification functions.

Another excellent exercise for your heart is a total-body, non- impact sport such astennis or squash, swimming or rowing, Tae Kwondo or other Martial Arts. All of these involve the use of many different muscles so give your body a good workout without overtaxing any one area, but making your heart work hard to supply them all. You can also create your own ideal workout that fits your current fitness level by incorporating slow intervals.

Core workouts such as push-ups and squats help to strengthen the core muscles, providing your body a good
64

foundation. People who are active all day long are generally healthier than those who exercise 30 minutes to an hour a day and live a sedentary lifestyle for the rest of the day. But bear in mind that not all exercises are good for the body. For instance, jogging or running on hard surfaces for long distance is probably the worst types of exercise although they do strengthen the heart. It's because such endurance-type exercises wear the body out quickly and strain your joints in the long term, especially if you don't have a pair or comfortable shoes or proper running techniques.

Equally, it is not advisable to perform any exercise that you have not trained or warmed up for. Doing so will only result in unwanted injuries and even trigger a heart attack due to adrenaline surge. If you have an exercise routine that you enjoy, then follow it and improve it by adding to it, rather than changing to something you may not enjoy.

Stress Reduction

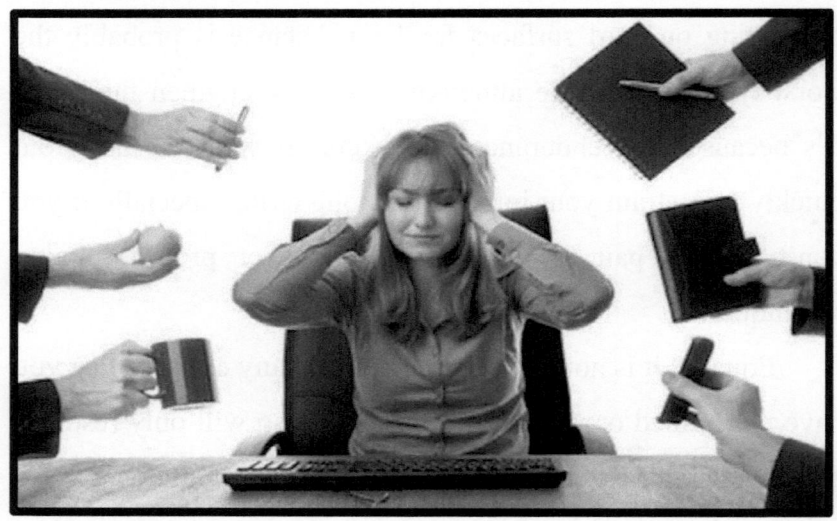

Countless studies prove that psychological factors can contribute to heart disease and possible heart attacks. Anxiety, anger, depression, hostility as well as social isolation can affect your heart attack risk factor.

Workplace stress and financial stress can increase your risk of a heart attack by 50%. After the 9/112001 terrorist attacks, it was found people who felt high levels of stress just after the attack were twice as likely to develop high blood pressure and had a threefold chance of developing develop heart disease over the following two years. Similar results have been observed after large earthquakes and other natural disasters.

Environmental Conditions, Clean Air and Water

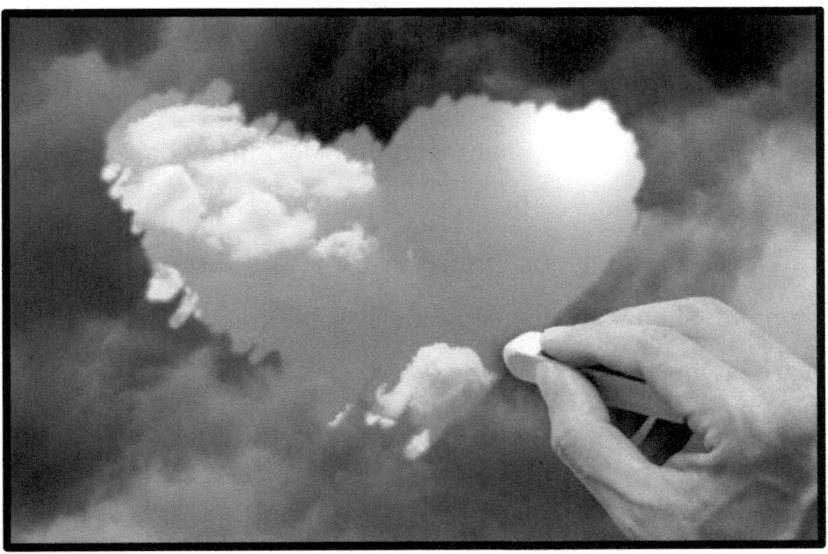

Water and air pollution are significant contributors to people developing heart disease and stroke (a stroke is like a heart attack to the brain). Staying indoor too often might not be as safe as you think because there's indoor air pollution.

Pollution comes from a mixture of different contaminants such as fumes from household cleaning products, wood burning stoves, and fireplaces, second-hand cigarette smoke, vapors from cleaning products, paint solvents, pesticides, insecticides and carbon monoxide.

Exposure to low levels of CO (Cardio Monoxide) can cause a cardiovascular patient to have increased heart rhythm, chest pain, and irregularities that make it difficult to exercise. Indoor CO can come from inside furnaces, dryers, gas water heaters, space heaters, ranges, and fireplace sand wood stoves.

There is evidence that several minerals commonly found in drinking water may contribute to heart disease or aggravate its symptoms. Lead, arsenic, fluoride and chlorine exposure are all clearly associated with heart disease.

CHAPTER 6

REMEDIES FOR A HEALTHY HEART

Many natural remedies use a variety of herbs and supplements to help treat as well as prevent heart disease. Atherosclerosis the hardening of the arteries is a common cause of heart disease. This disease is found mainly in the western world. On the other hand, atherosclerosis is relatively rare in the third world countries due to the difference in lifestyles, access to traditional diets and herb remedies. Most importantly, they're free from chemicals and toxins from the processed foods that can jeopardize the heart's health.

Coenzyme Q10, or ubiquinone, is a compound that helps our cells extract energy from food. This compound is often missing from our diets. Although Coenzyme Q10 is produced naturally in our body, the amount decreases dramatically as a person grows older or has reduced cholesterol levels. So by supplementing Coenzyme Q10 in your daily stack, you can ensure that your body has an adequate supply of nutrients to sustain your heart and keep your cells healthy.

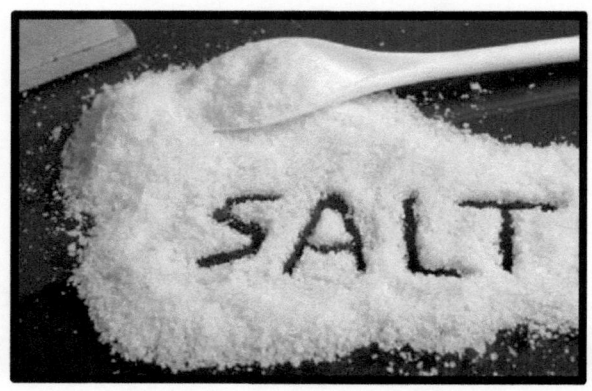

If you are not getting enough magnesium and potassium in your diet, by taking these supplements can help you regulate your blood pressure levels as well as improve heart function. As you may or may not know, salt goes a long way back in the human's history. It plays a vital role in both the development of human civilization as well as public health politics in the past centuries. Although salt was highly-regarded as a prized ingredient for thousands of years, it was demonized in the past century. Today, it was even named as one of the single most harmful substance in the human body.

However, recent studies have shown that although the amount of salt intake affects the heart health, it still plays a significant role in a healthy heart and optimal health. In fact, too little salt can cause various diseases and harm your body in the long run. Thus, we should consume salt in moderation for better health.

So where do we get our salt?

Natural, unrefined sea or rock salt are a great source of minerals.

Sea salt is the best source of salt that we can find to enrich our food with an abundance of minerals. Today, it's difficult to find a trace of healthy minerals in our food due to the shortage of nutrient-rich soil. So by adding a variety of sea salts to our food, we can obtain the much-needed minerals from the Earth's oceans.

But not all salts are good for our health. In fact, table salt which is mined from the salt deposits underground is heavily processed and detrimental to our health. Processed table salt is stripped of its natural minerals and often includes additive to avoid clumping.

You can only reap all the health benefits of the minerals from the ocean by choosing whole, natural sea salt that's "worth its salt". Not to mention the incredible taste that it can bring to your best dishes.

- **Fish Oil and other Supplements**

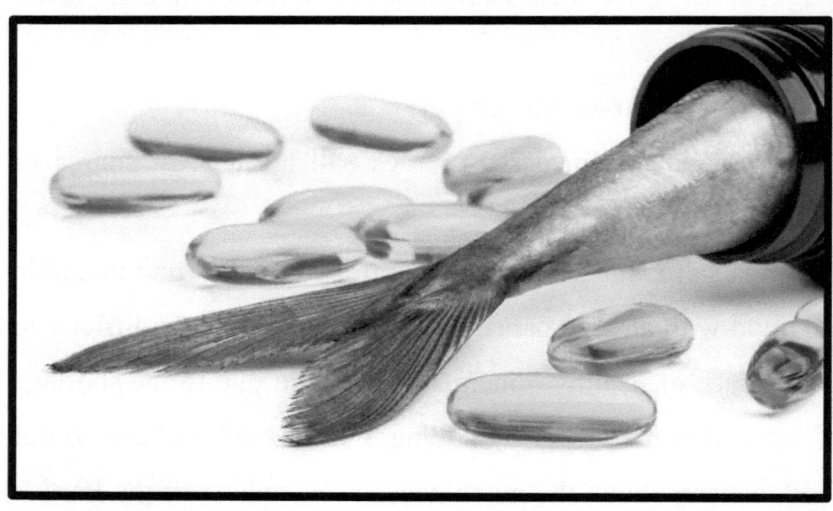

Many supplements like fish oil are often of low quality and can be harmful. This is due to the extraction process used which causes them to oxidize. It is important to access the quality before purchasing or taking any supplements. Typically, a good wholesome diet will supply all the needs of the body.

The only time supplements become necessary is when your diet is lacking or when certain health conditions cause you to develop an insufficiency or deficiency. Most dietary supplements are safe, and some of them offer actual health benefits, but there can be some risk with their use. Some of these are also anti-nutrients; they prevent the body absorbing nutrients.

Omega-3 Fatty Acids are essential nutrients that are found in naturally grown plants, free range, naturally fed livestock and sea caught fish. Usually, in nature, they are found in the ideal proportion for heart health of 50/50 with other natural fats such as omega-6 fats.

Livestock such as eggs, dairy and seafood lack many essential nutrients when they are raised in feedlots or factory farms without natural feeds or natural sunshine. They lack omega-3 fats and contain very high amount of damaging fats which is bad for health.

So if you're not consuming free-range organic food, then you're highly recommended to include supplements in your diet to fulfill your daily nutritional needs.

- **Vitamins and their Importance**

Health experts find that Vitamin C is undoubtedly one of the safest and much-needed nutrients for the human body. By taking in a daily dose of Vitamin C, your body will have a similar effect with walking. A simple exercise as walking can stimulate a protein known as endothelin-1, which induces the constriction of small blood vessels. Studies show that people who take a daily time- release dose of Vitamin C at 500 mg can inhibit the endothelin-1 activity as much as those who walkedregularly.

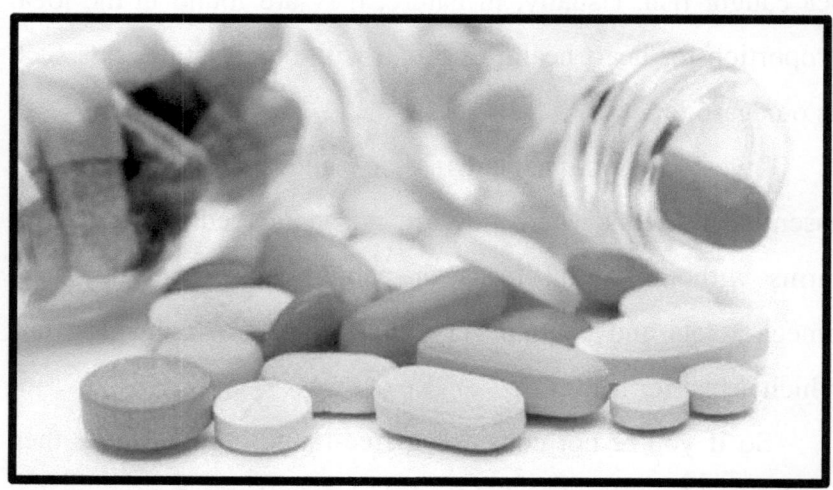

Vitamin B9, also known as folic acid is one the water-soluble vitamins. It's one of the essential vitamins that you should include in your daily nutritional needs. Our liver acts as a storage for vitamins.

On a daily basis, our body will utilize the required amount of vitamin from this storage. The excess amount of vitamins is then eliminated from our body automatically through the excretory system. Vitamin B9 aids in one of the most important functions of the body, which includes everything from the formation of red blood cells to the production of vital energy.

Besides that, Vitamin B9 also provides health benefits such as creating a defensive barrier from cancer, stroke, heart diseases, and birth anomalies. Other advantages include muscle building, haemoglobin formation, and also prevention from mental and emotional breakdowns. Vitamin B9 can be found naturally in asparagus, broccoli, Brussels sprouts, and lentils.

- **Enzymes in Foods**

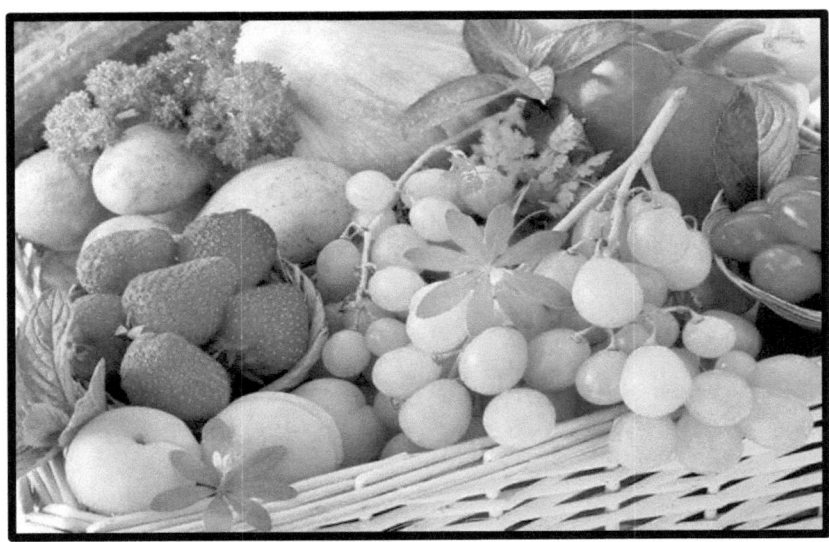

Enzymes are vital for every cell in our body as they are organic, biological catalyst that starts, promote and speed up biochemical reactions.

Metabolic enzymes in the blood break down the protein-based protection of virus' parasites, bacteria and fungi. They are cleansers that combat chronic inflammation, preventing most diseases including heart disease. Our body produces many enzymes; millions a day, but we still need a good supply of fresh enzymes from fresh food.

- **Antioxidants**

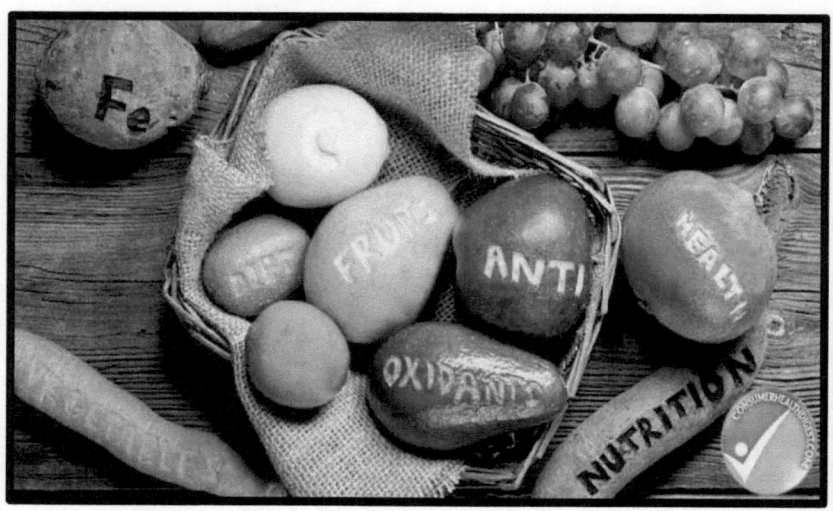

When you eat a healthy wholesome diet with plenty of raw, fresh fruits and vegetables, you get a good variety of enzymes and antioxidants as well as fiber.

Antioxidants are molecules that give off electrons that help to maintain the integrity of your cells. Antioxidants help to prevent cholesterol from oxidizing. In fact, oxidized cholesterol is the reason of fatality.

Although oxidation is one of the normal bodily processes, it can be life-threatening if there's an overproduction of oxidized cholesterol.

Why is that so? It's because unlike the other products of oxidation, oxidized cholesterol is commonly mistaken as bacteria by our natural immune system. Thus, your body will do whatever it takes to eliminate oxidized cholesterol from the body, causing inflammation of the arterial walls. As a result, it can lead to atherosclerosis or even heart diseases.

There are many recognized antioxidants, but the one of the most well-known is vitamin E. Study after study has shown that vitamin E is a potent antioxidant that can help prevent and even treat free radical damage.

- **Factory Farming VS Organic Foods**

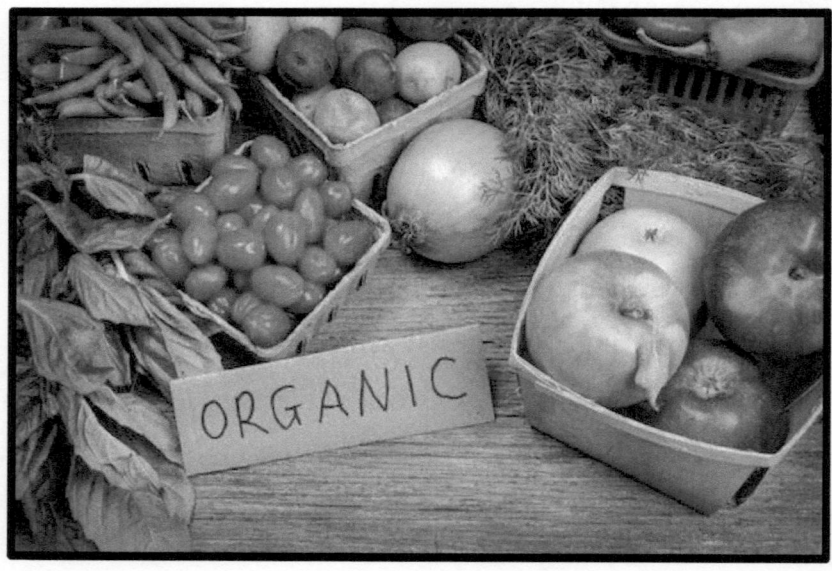

Have you heard of the term "Factory Farming"? It's a modern day term that refers to the "non-traditional" approach to farming businesses that focuses on keeping animals at high stocking densities. They're able to achieve this goal by incorporating modern technology to hasten animal growth, increase production outputs, and reduces the death rate of livestock.

The modern society, especially business owners and investors, share the same opinion that factory farming is the way to go for modern farming. Factory farming was also regarded as one of the top innovations and believed to solve countless issues, providing high production output and lowering the cost. On the other hand, there are also some who are against it, claiming that factory farming brings more harm than good to both our health and environment. Animal activists also protest against animal cruelty practices in factory farming.

So what is the truth?

After years of close monitoring and extensive studies in the agriculture sector, it is found that most factory farming utilize poor quality ingredients and questionable processing methods.

On the other hand, there's an "Organic" way of farming. This term refers to the more natural, less toxic approach on how the agricultural products are grown and produced. For instance, organic crops must be grown without the use of modern agricultural chemicals such as GMOs (Bioengineered genes), synthetic pesticides, sewage sludge-based, and petroleum based fertilizers.

Organic livestock must not be injected with growth hormones, antibiotics, or animal by-products. Organic livestock must be grown with organic feed and given access to roam outdoors. Any less than that cannot be labeled as "organic".

Thus, organic agricultural products are far more nutritional and less toxic to our body. Consuming more organic food and less factory-farmed food can lead to better health with more retained nutrients.

- **Detox - the real story**

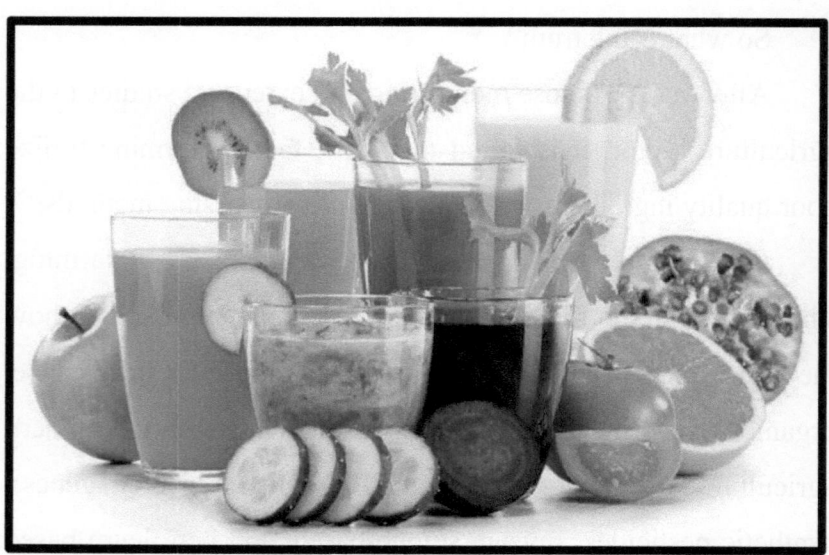

Our bodies, if given the raw materials needed are very good at detoxing themselves. People who have a healthy wholesome diet and refrains from indulging in too many processed foods (a small amount of processed food is not ideal, but the body can deal with it if not overloaded) will enjoy renewed energy and heart health.

- **Meditative Cures, Reflexology and Mindfulness**

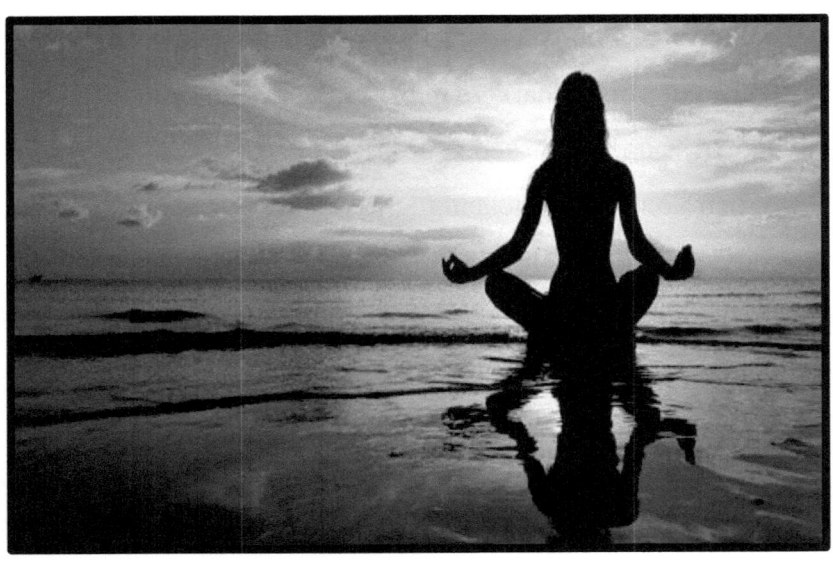

Psychological risk factors including anxiety and depression are clearly factors that can have a substantial effect on the heart.

Stress can affect and increase the risk factors for heart disease and high blood pressure (BP), especially if coupled with physical inactivity and a person being overweight.

Based on the latest clinical findings, it is found that meditation can drastically reduce the risk of heart diseases, stroke, and even death by approximately 50%. They found that deep breathing and acute relaxation can be more effective than any latest super drugs to prevent or even cure heart diseases.

The ultimate goal of meditation is to find "Balance" within our body. Although this may sound intangible and hard to grasp by the majority of our society today, meditation has been proven to balance out our biomarkers in the body. These biomarkers are also known as hormones and neurotransmitter.

When you're experiencing stress or pain from any part of the body, it's normally due to the hormonal changes and neurotransmitter imbalance. A powerful cure for this situation is meditation. This practice helped countless of patients to regulate their biomarkers.

Why is meditation so powerful? The secret lies in the practice of mindfulness.

Mindfulness is a term that refers to being able to focus your awareness on the present moment and everything around you, both internally and externally.

One of the keys of mindfulness is to always be at the present moment. Being present to your thoughts, emotions, and behaviors without judging them. The practice of non-judgement is the essence of staying truly calm and present.

The benefits of mindfulness are endless. Studies have demonstrated that people who practice mindfulness regularly are more likely to live longer, have healthier hearts, stronger immune system, and unlikely to be obese.

Another alternative therapy for heart health is reflexology.

This method appeals to those who seek for non-invasive therapy. In fact, some people might even find reflexology to be rather relaxing and therapeutic. It's not necessary to visit the reflexology centres to reap the benefits as you can easily apply these self-relaxing techniques yourself at any time on your hands and feet, provided that you know how to do it properly.

Reflexology helps to maintain the balance of the mind and body by keeping them in a homeostasis state, so that the body can function optimally. By applying pressure at certain pressure points of the body, trained reflexologists are able to fix the malfunctioned body and put your body in the natural equilibrium state.

Applying pressure at certain pressure points are able to stimulate your muscles, tissues, and even cells of any parts of your body. These pressure points are also known as reflexes on the hands and feet.

Different pressure points affect different parts of the body. In order to relax and invigorate the myocardial muscles, the pressure points are located on the reflexes on your feet, which also indirectly stimulates the colon and pituitary gland.

- **Super Foods for Heart Health**

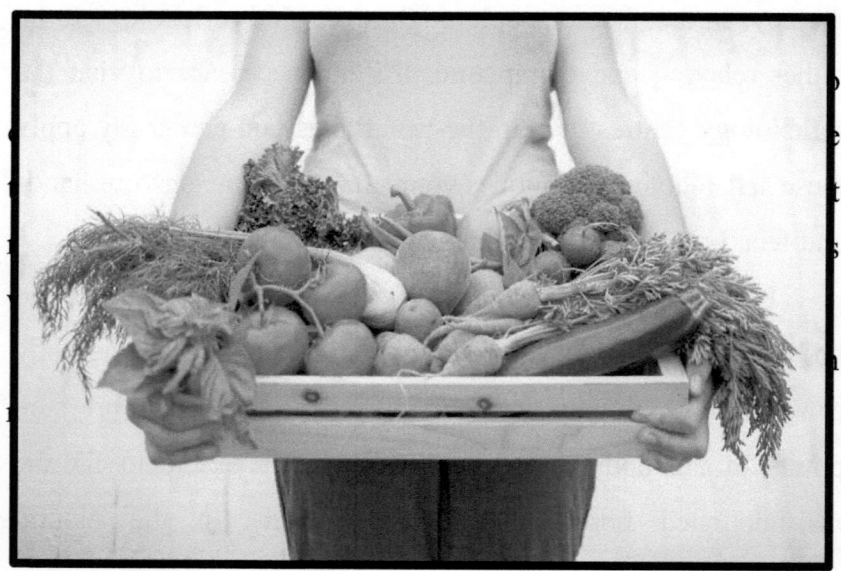

Asparagus has been found to be a very effective blood cleanser, it is able to reduce blood pressure and slow the forming of blood clots. It is loaded with Vitamins B1, B2, C, E and K.

Pomegranates have an impressive array of antioxidants that help to protect artery membranes; they also promote the production of nitric oxide that allows a person's blood to flow more freely through their blood vessels.

Turmeric reduces inflammation and the hardening of the arteries as well as helping to keep them clear and reduce blood clots.

Persimmon is a very good source of polyphenols and antioxidants that both help to reduce bad cholesterol (LDL) and triglycerides. They also help to normalize blood pressure and cleanse the arteries.

Spirulina helps to regulate blood fat levels, normalizes lipid levels and contains necessary essential amino acids, which help to improve the immune system.

Cinnamon is able to decrease harmful cholesterol levels and clean plaque so it is unable to accumulate in the arteries and blood vessels.

Broccoli helps to prevent calcium build up in arteries and helps to reduce blood pressure and normalize cholesterol levels.

Cranberries are thought to decrease the risk of developing heart disease in most people by up to 40%. They have a high antioxidant content which helps to increase HDL while reducing LDL levels.

Green Tea contains a large amount of catechins which help to decelerate the absorption of cholesterol and improve blood lipid levels as they help to clear obstructions from arteries. Green tea also helps with cardiovascular health and enhances a person's metabolism.

CONCLUSION

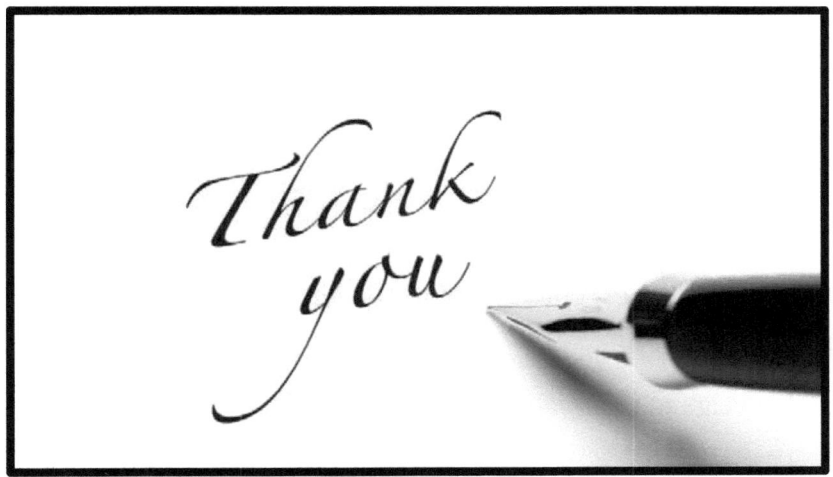

Thank you for purchasing this guidebook. I hope you enjoy this book and benefit immensely from it.

As a general rule, our body's overall health starts with taking care of our heart. If you are looking after your heart, then you will also be looking after the rest of your body. The decisions that you make regarding your diet and lifestyle will ultimately affect your heart health, your overall wellbeing. Not just that, your family will also be affected.

If you're following a diet that consists of mainly processed foods, you're putting poisons into your body with empty carbohydrates and chemicals. Plus, if you're inactive in most parts of the day and live a sedentary lifestyle, you can expect to have major health issues at some point in your life, and you'll ultimately reduce your lifespan.

On the other hand, if you have a healthy lifestyle, take sensible precautions on your food intake, and are active in physical exercises; then you can expect to live a long, healthy life, free of heart problems and many other chronic health issues that plague most people. This will allow you to enjoy your golden years in relatively good health.

Printed by Libri Plureos GmbH in Hamburg, Germany

9 786069 836903